Other books by Cathy Covell

A Therapist's Guide to Understanding
Myofascial Release

Feeling Your Way Through

A Patient's Guide to Understanding Myofascial Release

Simple Answers to Frequently Asked Questions

Cathy Covell

BALBOA.
PRESS
A DIVISION OF HAY HOUSE

Balboa Press books may be ordered through booksellers or by contacting:

Balboa Press
A Division of Hay House
1663 Liberty Drive
Bloomington, IN 47403
www.balboapress.com
1 (877) 407-4847

Because of the dynamic nature of the Internet, any web addresses or
links contained in this book may have changed since publication and
may no longer be valid. The views expressed in this work are solely those
of the author and do not necessarily reflect the views of the publisher,
and the publisher hereby disclaims any responsibility for them.

The author of this book does not dispense medical advice or prescribe
the use of any technique as a form of treatment for physical, emotional,
or medical problems without the advice of a physician, either directly
or indirectly. The intent of the author is only to offer information
of a general nature to help you in your quest for emotional and
spiritual well-being. In the event you use any of the information in
this book for yourself, which is your constitutional right, the author
and the publisher assume no responsibility for your actions.

Any people depicted in stock imagery provided by Thinkstock are
models, and such images are being used for illustrative purposes only.
Certain stock imagery © Thinkstock.

Printed in the United States of America.

ISBN: 978-1-4525-8957-2 (sc)
ISBN: 978-1-4525-8958-9 (e)

Balboa Press rev. date: 1/3/2014

Contents

Special Thanks!!

First and foremost thanks to John F. Barnes, PT! If it weren't for you, none of this would be possible. There aren't enough words to express everything you have done for me by being strong enough to follow your intuition. Thanks for your love and your guidance.

Thanks to Valerie McGraw and Carol Bannister for your support with this book. Carol, thanks for helping me when I couldn't quite put what I was thinking into writing. Val, thanks for your endless supply of faith in my ability and for your support during the times I hit the stumbling blocks. You were a rock during the storms.

Thanks to Sandy Hilton for being a sounding board, an editor, and a resource into the world of publishing. Thanks also to Dave and Jan Frederick. I really appreciate all the help.

Thanks to Donna Killion for your compassion and support during my healing process. You've helped me more than you know.

And a big thanks to all the people in the John F. Barnes' Myofascial Release (JFB-MFR) community who encouraged me to put my MFR chat posts together in one book.

About This Edition

This edition of *A Patient's Guide to Understanding Myofascial Release* contains updated information, rewritten material, and corrections to copy errors in the previous edition. I worked closely with Joe Miller, LCMT, in producing this edition. Joe suggested manuscript and copy edits to the original edition of this book; I accepted the ones I felt maintained my original meaning and tone.

Joe brought a special combination of abilities to the editing of this edition. A licensed, nationally-certified massage therapist practicing JFB-MFR exclusively, Joe began his journey with JFB-MFR at the Healing Seminar in 2002. He has practiced JFB-MFR exclusively since 2004.

Before becoming a massage therapist in order to practice JFB-MFR, Joe spent over 25 years as a professional writer, editor, and business and technical consultant to companies in the United States and Europe. His knowledge of writing and editing, of JFB-MFR, and of collaborative work methods helped me make significant improvements in this new edition.

Joe practices JFB-MFR in the Chicago area. He also continues to write, edit, and provide language translation services to clients. You can reach Joe at jlmsvcs@gmail.com.

Forward

John F. Barnes' Myofascial Release is the ultimate therapeutic art. Therapists and patients first learn the work on a structural level. As they progress in treatment, they find great depth to the JFB-MFR approach. As skills and senses sharpen, the therapist and patient become aware of physical, emotional, mental, and energetic levels. It is at these levels that true healing can occur, creating large shifts in overall health. The best results are seen with those who have had the courage to delve deeply into their own healing possibilities and to take leaps out of their comfort zone.

Cathy Covell is one of those therapists who have dared to explore the possibilities of healing. She has come through her own pain to find techniques that affect real change. Cathy worked for me at the Paoli Myofascial Release Treatment Center and is a great therapist. The Myofascial Release Seminars teach therapists from all over the world a technique that truly has the best interest of the patient at heart. Cathy has excelled in Myofascial Release and has been instrumental in answering questions on the Myofascial Release Chat Line with clarity while also keeping with the principles of true Myofascial Release.

The examples and insights provided in this book offer help to people during their healing journey. Reading and re-reading this book—as well as reading my book *Healing Ancient Wounds: The Renegade's Wisdom*, and watching my videos *The Fireside Chat* and the MFR DVD set—will enable people to understand the JFB-MFR process at an even deeper level.

I hope you read the examples in this book slowly and carefully, and approach the questions posed here with the intention of seeing yourself in a new light. Read the question at the beginning of each chapter and pay attention to your reaction to the response to that question. See if you have a particular resistance to self-treatment, or emotion, or unwinding. See if you can go more deeply into the feeling and move past your own restrictions to a new quality of life and health. Learning is a life-long process; it does not end. It is important to enjoy the journey. This book is a valuable tool in helping you along the way.

John F. Barnes, PT
President of the Myofascial Release Treatment Centers and Seminars
1-800-Fascial
www.myofascialrelease.com

Introduction

The two books *A Patient's Guide to Understanding Myofascial Release* and *A Therapist's Guide to Understanding Myofascial Release* came together as a surprise for me. If I hadn't been given quite firm encouragement by some fellow therapists and friends, these books might not have been published. Just for my own benefit, I started collecting these answers to questions I heard frequently; then they turned into chapters and books.

While working at John Barnes' Myofascial Release Treatment Center in Paoli, PA[1], I was asked frequently the questions that have become the chapter titles in this book. I started saving my responses to many of those questions so I could refer to them as needed; this book is a compilation of those responses. The questions came from patients at the Paoli Clinic, from patients receiving JFB-MFR at other facilities, and from people considering getting treatment. Some of the questions were asked on the MFR chat line. Anyone can join the free chat line on John's website (www.myofascialrelease. com) and ask questions or share information. This book

---

[1]   The Myofascial Release Treatment Center in Paoli, PA has since been relocated to a facility in Malvern, PA.

is a direct result of my posts on the MFR chat line, my daily interaction with patients and other therapists, my own journey of breaking free of chronic pain, and my listening to and learning from John.

Two invaluable resources are John's DVD *The Fireside Chat* and his MFR DVD set. *The Fireside Chat*, a 75-minute discussion with John, provides an inside look at John's perspective on the principles and methods employed in his Myofascial Release Approach. This DVD was designed to help therapists and patients understand the Myofascial Release philosophy on a deeper level. It can also help your loved ones understand the possibilities of a better life through the MFR process.

My book gives general answers and explanations to some of the questions patients and therapists ask most frequently when considering or receiving JFB-MFR treatment. For more thorough discussions of how JFB-MFR was developed and of the healing process, read John's book *Healing Ancient Wounds: The Renegade's Wisdom*.

I hope the information in this book is easy to understand and helps you with your healing process. Enjoy the journey. Believe me, it's worth it!

My background with JFB-MFR

My road to discovering the benefits of JFB-MFR involved my own physical pain and dysfunction. I know having my own pain has helped me become a much better therapist.

Many of my symptoms began to manifest while I was in high school. I began having problems with ovarian cysts and had at least one ovarian cyst rupture each year through my late 20s. During my junior year in college, I had surgery to remove my right ovary and a large cyst. After I graduated with my first degree and before starting physical therapy school, I began having back pain.

I have played sports all of my life. In college, I played volleyball and basketball and was used to having a very active lifestyle. As my pain continued to increase, I was unable to walk more than a few blocks before I had to stop because of pain down my leg and spasms in my back. I thought surgery was my only option, so that is what I did. I underwent surgery in May and started physical therapy school in August. After the surgery, I didn't have constant numbness, but I still had pain, spasms, and occasional numbness.

During physical therapy school, and for the five years after I graduated, I searched for a way to relieve my own pain. I tried everything I was taught in school, with little result, and then started taking continuing education classes. I focused on taking any seminar having to do with the pelvis or the back. I tried all the manipulations, mobilizations, stabilization exercises, and stretches that were supposed to help alleviate back pain. I was unable to find anything that gave me more than temporary relief.

Believe me, it was very frustrating to be a physical therapist that was in more pain than her patients. I was also frustrated that many of my patients continued to have pain after receiving treatment. I felt like there was something I was missing. So, I started trying alternative treatments. I had about every kind of massage available and also tried acupuncture. All produced only temporary benefits.

My good days were ones when I had a constant dull ache; my bad days were when my leg would go numb or I had a knife-like pain in my back. I was unable to sit or stand for more than 20–30 seconds without needing to shift my weight due to the pain. I was slowly giving up the things I loved to do, like playing sports and riding horses. I was told that my pain was due to scar tissue and there was really nothing that could be done to help with scar tissue.

Here I was, in my mid- to late-20s and in constant pain. I didn't even want to think about what life would be like when I reached my 50s. It was very depressing and frustrating.

It was at this time a therapist colleague offered to treat me using JFB-MFR. Honestly, I didn't really have much faith it would help, but I thought I would just go along with it. I didn't have anything to lose by trying.

Within three or four treatments I felt a significant change for the better. I will always remember the night I lay down in bed and was able to straighten my legs fully. Previously, I always had to sleep with my knees bent and my trunk turned to the side or else I would have too much pain. My first thought was, "Wow, I can put my legs straight without pain!" Then my second thought was, "Well, we'll see how long this lasts." I was so used to having temporary results I didn't think these results wouldn't last either. Well, it's been over five years now and I'm still sleeping with my legs straight!

To say JFB-MFR has given me my life back is an understatement. I can honestly say that I feel better at 36 than I did at 26. Not only that, but I now have the knowledge to help keep my body in the best shape possible for the rest of my life.

After my first treatments, I signed up to take classes taught by John Barnes. I wanted to be able to help others the way I was helped. The classes opened up my life professionally as well as personally. I finally learned ways to help patients heal themselves. The whole body approach taught by John completely changed the way I treated as a therapist.

I continued to take John's classes and also participated in a Skill Enhancement Seminar at his Paoli, Pennsylvania Myofascial Release Treatment Center. This led to getting a position as a coverage therapist at Paoli and eventually led into working full time at the Treatment Center for 2 ½ years.

Being able to work at John's Paoli Clinic was a huge catalyst in both my personal and professional growth. The experience I received helped me gain the confidence needed to start teaching a seminar on treating horses using JFB-MFR.

In 2007, I returned to my home in Indiana so I could be close to my family and bring JFB-MFR to the area. I continue to work as a coverage therapist in the Paoli Treatment Center, help at John's seminars, and teach an Equine seminar.

Every day I am thankful John followed his intuition in developing these techniques and shares his knowledge with others. I hope this book helps you have a better understanding of JFB-MFR so you can progress along your path to healing like I have done.

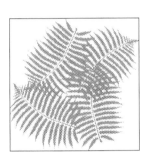

1
What is JFB-MFR?

I am about to give a very quick and limited explanation of John F. Barnes' Myofascial Release (JFB-MFR). To get a more thorough understanding of JFB-MFR, please refer to the many articles and books John has written. In these you will find the references to and scientific rational for true myofascial release. In this book, I hope to give you a basic understanding of myofascial release.

True JFB-MFR is a full-body, hands-on technique developed and refined by John F. Barnes, PT. This technique releases the fascial system, a three-dimensional web connecting and surrounding every system and cell in the body. To help people get the idea of the role of the fascial system, I like to compare the human body to an orange.

Outer layer: The thick, white, hard tissue that attaches an orange to the peel is similar to the fascia that holds the skin to our body.

Inner layer: When you cut an orange in half, the white fibers separate the different chambers of the orange. Fascia in our body helps to separate our organs and keep them in place. If it didn't, when we stood up, all our organs would drop down into our legs!

Cellular layer: When you look at an individual orange slice, you see the white fibers weaving throughout the slice, holding the slice together and also holding in the juice. Again, this is very similar to the fascial system holding our bodies together down to the cellular level. Our bodies are over 70% fluid and the fascial system is what keeps all this fluid (along with all the vital organs, nerves, veins, and arteries) in the right place.

Through trauma and repetitive motion or positioning (lifting all day or sitting all day), restrictions can form in the fascial system. These restrictions can exert forces up to 2000 pounds per square inch. This force can literally crush any of the vital structures near it. Since the fascial system runs throughout your entire body, these restrictions can cause pain anywhere in the body and compromise any system.

By "system," I mean vascular, neurological, muscular, reproductive, circulatory, digestive, etc. Fascial restrictions can cause digestive problems, fertility problems, circulation problems, neurological problems, cellular problems, muscular problems, etc.

These restrictions can become tighter over time, leaving you feeling like you are in a straitjacket and sending symptoms throughout your body.

JFB-MFR helps to remove the straitjacket from the body. A skilled therapist looks at and treats the entire body, helping to restore balance. Releasing the fascial restrictions throughout the body decreases the crushing force of fascial restrictions, which in turn increases function, decreases pain, increases blood flow and nutrition to the body, and increases overall health down to the cellular level.

Fascial restrictions cannot be seen by x-ray or any other standard imaging technology. However, by developing sensitivity through taking courses and being treated, a skilled JFB-MFR therapist can see and feel where these fascial restrictions are located. A JFB-MFR treatment consists of engaging the barrier of the restriction and then waiting, allowing the restriction to release.

The barrier is the point at which the fascial restriction is in a lengthened or slightly stretched position. This is different from the end range of motion; it's more like taking the slack out of the system. Once the therapist engages the restriction at the barrier, it then needs to be held there for a minimum of 90-120 seconds before it **starts** to release.

For a good release to occur, the restriction needs to be held at the barrier at least 3-5 minutes. If the therapist holds the restriction at the barrier for a shorter time, he is not doing authentic JFB-MFR and is not allowing the tissue to make a permanent change. Anything less does not involve the collagen component and works on only the elastic part—fascia is roughly 80% collagen and 20% elastic— and provides only temporary relief.

True JFB-MFR is not forceful. The body is allowed to release, not forced to release. This does not mean the releases will not be painful. Pain and many other sensations often occur during a release. This is described more completely in the following chapters. To receive true JFB-MFR, you need to be treated by a therapist who works according to the following guidelines:

- looks at and treats the entire body;
- engages the barrier and does not force though the barrier;
- holds at the barrier for at least 3-5 minutes to allow for a true release to occur;
- does not force or lead; and
- does not interpret what you are feeling. Each person's experience is unique to him or her.

If your therapy is not done by following these guidelines, your therapist may not fully understand the principles of JFB-MFR. Some therapists take one or two classes from John—or take a class in school—and believe they are doing JFB-MFR, but they don't fully understand the key principles. It's okay to question your therapists. If you have concerns, remember you can always voice them on John's MFR chat line, located on his website at: www.myofascialrelease.com. This is a nice support system and a really good way to have questions answered and concerns addressed.

So, get ready for your adventure with JFB-MFR. If you are looking for true, authentic healing, you have come to the right place!

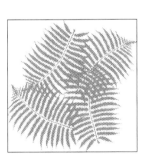

2

How is JFB-MFR different from other forms of therapy?

There are a number of significant differences between JFB-MFR and other types of bodywork and traditional therapies. Other forms of bodywork and therapies generally do not follow what the body needs. They follow protocols and are what can be called "cookbook techniques." Many treat only symptoms, try to segment the body, and ignore the power of the consciousness.

JFB-MFR is a whole body approach that engages the fascia and follows what the body needs. JFB-MFR therapists tune into what each individual needs by engaging the barrier of the restriction and waiting for the release to occur. This is a key difference between JFB-MFR and other forms of bodywork.

Neither traditional nor alternative therapies hold at the barrier for sufficient time and therefore release only the elastic and muscular component of the myofascial complex. This is why these forms of therapy provide only temporary results. The JFB-MFR approach releases the collagenous aspect of the myofascial complex, bringing about lasting results. The restriction needs to be held at the barrier for at least 3-5 minutes to allow the collagen to lengthen.

To illustrate this point, I like to compare two ways of stretching a rubber band. If you stretch a rubber band between your fingers, it lengthens. If you release the stretch after about a minute, the rubber band goes back to its original shape. This is like those therapies which hold at the barrier for only 30-45 seconds: all that is produced is a temporary result. You may feel relief for a little while, but then you feel that old familiar pull and pain again.

If you stretch that same rubber band around an object like a book and leave it for several minutes, it will have lengthened when you remove it. This is what JFB-MFR does: causes a permanent lengthening of the tissue. These rubber band stretching examples make it easy to see the difference resulting from holding the stretch for several minutes and to realize the difference in effectiveness is massive. Go ahead—try it and see!

The awareness cultivated and used by JFB-MFR therapists is another big difference between JFB-MFR and other types of bodywork and traditional therapies. Feeling a restriction and holding the restriction at the barrier both require awareness. This barrier changes during the treatment as the fascia starts to release. The therapist needs to stay focused and centered to be able to feel the changes in the barrier, keeping at the barrier to keep the system engaged. If too much force is applied, the body starts to resist. If not enough force is applied, change occurs only in the elastic component, producing only temporary results.

It takes a therapist who is aware and centered to be able to maintain the barrier as the fascia releases. This is why it's important that the therapist who treats you has been taught at John F. Barnes' seminars. This awareness and feel cannot be learned through a book. This is also why some therapists are better qualified than others. Some therapists have gone to John's courses but are not able to stay centered. This makes it difficult or even impossible to feel the subtle changes that occur during a release.

True JFB-MFR is non-injurious, results in permanent changes, and can help a person heal in mind, body, and spirit. The reason JFB-MFR is non-injurious is due to the therapist's awareness during a treatment, to the therapist's ability to feel and not force the barrier.

This is also what allows the full healing capability of the body to occur. The reason JFB-MFR can help a person heal in mind and spirit is because the consciousness is recognized and enhanced. The awareness of the patient is very important in the healing process. This awareness is described more thoroughly in chapters 9 and 15, on feeling under the pain and on feeling emotions. All of these aspects taken together are why JFB-MFR is called authentic healing.

3

Can JFB-MFR help with…?

Many of the questions that come up at the seminars, on the chat line, and in the clinic start with "Can JFB-MFR help with [some diagnosis or another]?" At times therapists and patients both get caught up on the diagnosis. It seems the more specific or wordy a diagnosis, the more we doubt our ability to treat it. "I know JFB-MFR is a whole body treatment, but can it really help with spondylolysis of levels L2-4 with radiating sciatica and plantar fasciitis?" I mean, surely with a diagnosis that long, it would take more than "look at the body and see where it guides you."

A diagnosis is just a naming of the symptoms. It is just a way to fit symptoms into a category so they can be "treated" or "fixed." The only problem is, as soon as the label is put on a dysfunction, the person with the dysfunction is already being sold short. What

I mean is, when we as therapists or patients are given a diagnosis, our attention usually shifts to "How can I fix that?" instead of "Where am I, or where is the patient, restricted, or out of balance?" This shift causes a narrow focus which in turn limits results.

Can JFB-MFR help with every diagnosis? Yes it can. Am I saying that JFB-MFR can cure every diagnosis? No, I'm not. But, as John frequently says, freeing the body from restrictions will allow it to function more efficiently, often correcting itself. Not only does this work with acute dysfunctions like back trauma from falls, motor vehicle accidents, etc., but also with systemic and chronic diagnoses such as high blood pressure, diabetes, fibromyalgia, chronic fatigue syndrome, and depression. JFB-MFR can help those with chronic conditions peel back not only the physical restrictions, but also the emotions that hold the straitjacket in place.

Then there is the category of nerve/neural diagnosis: stroke, carpal tunnel syndrome, sciatica, etc. If the nerve has been completely severed, JFB-MFR will not restore the nerve function. But again, JFB-MFR can free the system so the available muscle activity will be more efficient. Remember each nerve is surrounded by and goes through fascia. A fascial restriction can pinch or crush the nerve, causing numbness, tingling, and other nerve symptoms.

Myofascial restrictions can simulate every symptom. Restrictions can compress muscles, nerves, and the components of every other system in the body. Age doesn't matter; you are never too young or too old to benefit from JFB-MFR. So, what have you got to lose except some restrictions?

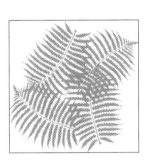

4

Will JFB-MFR overstretch the tissue?

Some people with hypermobility believe they must not have any restrictions. Others are concerned JFB-MFR could overstretch tissue. Hypermobility does not mean a person is free from restrictions; his or her body will still need to be balanced.

By really understanding the nature of JFB-MFR, you will realize true JFB-MFR cannot overstretch or tear tissue. Remember the principle of taking the fascia to the barrier and then holding it there. This allows the fascia to release; it is not forceful. To overstretch or damage tissue, a lot of force must be applied. Think of the rubber band example I used earlier. It takes a lot of force to cause a rubber band to break. You have to stretch it way past its barrier and all the way to the breaking point. Or, think of the amount of force required to pull a muscle. Usually a muscle gets pulled when a lot of force is applied with a lot of velocity, like pulling a hamstring muscle when sprinting or stopping quickly. JFB-MFR therapists are taught not to force the barrier, so when the therapist follows the guidelines, there is no way to overstretch or tear the tissue.

JFB-MFR helps restore elasticity to the tissue by breaking down the scar tissue and adhesions that can form through trauma or repetitive positioning. Restoring this elasticity or "give" in the system actually will help prevent injuries. This "give" allows tissue to absorb impacts and to stretch instead of breaking when force is applied. Think of recurring sprains and strains. Why does the same area keep getting injured? After each injury, more scar tissue forms in the area to help prevent movement during healing. With more scar tissue, this area has even less ability to absorb impact or to stretch under force and so it tears again under impact or other force. Releasing the restrictions in such an area will allow the tissue to heal and help prevent re-injury.

5

Why is my therapist treating areas other than where the symptoms are located?

Many doctors, therapists, and other health professionals are taught to treat symptom areas as a way to "fix" a patient's dysfunction. This seems like a good approach, but it really has not proved to be particularly effective. Instead of being taught to treat symptoms, the medical profession should be looking for the cause of the problem. Treating the symptoms—or masking them—doesn't help a person heal. It only gives temporary relief, if any relief at all. If the philosophy of treating the symptom worked, people would be returning to a functional lifestyle without being medicated. Instead, people often receive a prescription for medication to mask the pain or dysfunction, and frequently live in a drug-clouded reality as a result.

The JFB-MFR philosophy is to look at the entire being, instead of just focusing on where the symptoms are located. Many schools also teach this same philosophy to doctors and therapists. However, managed care insurance systems have focused on isolated body parts, contrary to the true tradition of medicine.

The area where the pain is expressing itself is often the weak point in the system and not where the actual problem originates. For example, suppose your pelvis is out of alignment. This dysfunction would cause the rest of your spine to be pulled off center. Your body wants to be upright, so your trunk and neck will try to counteract the pelvic misalignment, resulting in a scoliotic curve.

When the spine is in its natural alignment, the muscles along the spine are not very active. This is known as the position of rest or position of efficiency. These muscles can rest when your spine is in its natural position. When the spine is out of alignment, the muscles along your spine and neck have to work continuously and do not get to rest. This can cause soreness, pain, and muscle tension in these areas.

If you see your doctor because of this condition, you usually get a diagnosis which fits the symptoms, like neck pain, shoulder pain, or low back pain/strain. If you then go to a therapist, the therapist usually treats only your symptoms, giving you only temporary relief or sometimes actually making the symptoms worse. The only way you will truly heal is to receive treatment for the cause of the problem: the pelvic dysfunction.

Any diagnosis can have many different causes. Suppose you have shoulder pain. The pain might be due to an actual shoulder injury; it might be due to your pelvis being out of alignment; it might be due to an old knee injury; it might be due to any number of causes. The only way to know is to look at the entire body as a whole, and to help restore balance to the entire system.

As you receive JFB-MFR treatments, you will start to feel the whole body connection during the treatment. When you are being treated, let yourself sink into the area being treated and soon you will feel sensations in other parts of your body too. As your leg is being pulled, you may feel it in your hip and even up into your head or jaw. It's quite amazing when you start to feel this. After you start to feel the connections, you'll realize the body cannot be divided into segments. You will be able to feel the full-body, three-dimensional web of the fascial system.

Remember this connection as you do your self-treatment sessions. It's okay to start by treating the areas that are hurting. While you are treating those areas, let yourself feel where they connect. This is the area you will treat next. Your body will actually tell you where you need to treat (see chapter 18, *Can I treat myself?*). Let go of any ideas about where you need to be treated. Allow your body to guide you and you will get the treatment you need.

6

What if my symptoms get worse?

When your signs and symptoms become worse, you are experiencing what we call a "healing crisis." Sometimes this experience can feel just as intense as it did when you had the original injury, illness, or whatever else caused the symptoms. Why does this happen? One reason is that when you increase your awareness, you feel how much pain is actually there. Most of us have tuned out some of the pain. With increased awareness, you are now feeling the pain fully. This increase in signs and symptoms is your body's way of bringing your awareness to the condition with which you are dealing every day, a condition you "tune out" and don't feel.

Another reason a healing crisis occurs is that you are getting into the deeper layers of the restrictions. As you go deeper into the restrictions, you get closer to the most sensitive areas. This is the process we compare to peeling back the layers, like the layers of an onion. As you get into the deeper layers, not only might the symptoms intensify, but other sensations or emotions might also surface.

Typically, the healing crisis lasts 24–48 hours after a treatment, but it can continue longer. At times, it can feel like you are taking two steps forward and one step backwards. Just remember the healing process isn't a linear one. There will be ups and downs; this is normal.

It can be very scary when your body goes into a healing crisis. Remember JFB-MFR is never injurious. Using the self-treatment techniques your therapist taught you will help during this process. A regular self-treatment program, combined with your therapy sessions, will help speed your healing process.

It also helps to spend some quiet time bringing awareness into your body. Try to sink deeper into whatever feelings come up. Let yourself feel your symptoms fully and get in touch with what lies underneath. Give your body permission to let go of anything no longer serving you, and give yourself permission to do and feel whatever you need in order to heal.

As you tune in, you may experience memories, emotions, shaking, sweating...the list could go on and on. The key is to let yourself feel without any judgment or holding back. Allowing yourself to feel whatever comes up fully and letting it clear is a key component to the healing process. Sometimes the purpose of these "flare ups" is to help us tap into something—an emotion, a belief, an awareness—that needs to be felt so the restriction can release and healing can occur at a deeper level.

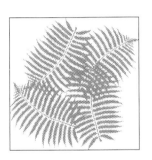

7

What happens when my original symptoms are better, but now I feel symptoms somewhere new?

After receiving treatment for a while, you may notice you are feeling "new" symptoms. For instance, your back doesn't seem to be hurting as much, but now your legs are suddenly very tight. Or, your neck pain is feeling better, but now you have shoulder pain. Does this mean you have new problems?

What is happening is you are peeling away the superficial layers away and progressing toward the deeper layers. When your most prevalent symptoms start to fade (and this is a good thing!), you will start to notice the other symptoms which were not significant enough to override your major symptom. I'll illustrate this using the examples from the beginning of this chapter.

The tightness in your legs was actually always there and was probably a result of bracing against your back pain. Your legs were tense and tight to help guard and protect your back. Now that your back has started to release, the tightness in your legs has become much more noticeable. The same thing is true for the neck and shoulder pain example. Once your neck starts to free up, the tightness and bracing in your shoulder becomes "louder."

When you start noticing these "new" pains, use it as an indication of improvement. The area formerly the most restricted, the most "loud," has released enough that now you can feel other areas in your body. Celebrate your feeling new symptoms as a sign of progress. Your body is telling you where you need to treat next.

The next step would be to treat these new areas and see where they lead you. If your original symptoms seem to become "loud" again, then you have once again reached a deeper level. You will start to realize the healing process is really quite simple. If you ever wonder where you need to treat, just ask your body!

8

Why is it when my therapist is treating one area I feel sensations in another area?

When I hear a sentence start with "This is weird, but..." I know the patient is starting to have increased body awareness. You may be feeling shaking, trembling, emotions, or other sensations. All of these are good developments and what we call becoming aware of the fascial voice. You are feeling the whole body connection and also the mind/body connection of the fascial system. John suggests we use the word "interesting" instead of "weird" because what is happening is actually normal. People associate the word "weird" with something they shouldn't be feeling because it's a word used to judge what they are feeling. The word "interesting" comes more from a place of curiosity.

The body is completely connected with a three-dimensional web of connective tissue called fascia. When your therapist is treating your neck, you may feel a response or connection in one of your toes. Or when your leg is being pulled, you may feel a connection all the way into your jaw. When you start to feel these connections, you may think it's "weird." Why is that? Because you have probably been told over and over that the body is not connected. Many doctors and therapists have been told this and that's what they tell their patients. Initially, when you start to feel the truth—that the whole body is actually connected—you may doubt what you are feeling or think you shouldn't be feeling the connection.

Feeling these connections is a vital part of the healing process. When you start to feel the connections, bring even more of your awareness in the areas being treated. (See chapter 9, *What does my therapist mean by "feel under the pain"?*). Once you start to feel the sensations or connections, allow yourself to feel them even more fully. When you feel sensations in an area other than the one being treated directly, this is the fascial voice talking. Your body is pointing out other areas that need treatment. By tuning in and listening to this inner guide, you are able to help yourself heal. The concepts of the fascial voice and of tuning in to see where to treat are an important part of your self-treatment.

The next time you find yourself starting a sentence with the words "This is weird...", recognize that you are probably on your way to reaching a new level of awareness. So, prepare yourself, because the fun is getting ready to start!

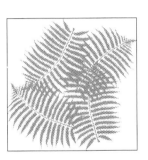

9

What does my therapist mean by "feel under the pain"?

Over the years, most of us have learned to tune out pain or other uncomfortable sensations. To really get the most benefit out of JFB-MFR treatments, you are going to need to do the opposite—allow yourself to feel all the sensations even more, including the unpleasant sensations. These sensations can include burning, aching, tearing, dull or sharp pains, tingling, and shaking, among many other possibilities.

When a sensation is painful or uncomfortable, you will need to "feel under the pain." You will help yourself do this by realizing that pain and other sensations are just signals and nothing else. Don't judge a sensation such as pain as "good" or "bad;" instead, just let it be what it is: a sensation. When you feel a sensation, instead of tuning it out, let yourself feel it even more. Feeling the sensation is what your body needs you to do so it can heal. Sensations are actually signals from your body.

When you feel a painful or uncomfortable sensation, your body is trying to bring your attention to an area in distress. It's trying to ask for help. When you don't listen to the more subtle signals—for instance, pressure or tightness—then it sends the louder signals—for instance, pain or achiness. When you tune into a sensation fully, you can start to help your body heal the area experiencing the sensation.

Pain is just a signal. Its job is similar to that of a smoke detector; in both cases, an alarm system tells us something is happening which needs our awareness. The only thing a smoke detector can do is tell us there is smoke. It doesn't tell us whether some toast is burning (a mild problem) or the house is on fire (a major problem!). All it does is send out a signal, and then it's up to us to go see what is wrong.

Pain is similar. It is a signal that tells us there is something we need to check out. What we need to do is acknowledge the signal, and then go see what needs to be done. Feel the pain and ask the body what it needs to do. Sometimes, all the body needs is our awareness and permission to let go. Other times, we may need to make a change—stop the activity we are doing, self-treat, unwind, etc. (Regarding unwinding, see chapter 17, *Why is my body moving?*)

Many of us have been taught to ignore our pain or just to treat the symptom (block the pain). That would be like going up to the smoke detector and putting a pillow over it. Yes, you are blocking out the noise and keeping the smoke from getting to the detector, but you may then find yourself caught in a burning house!

When you feel pain, remember it is just a signal. Try not to judge it. Let yourself really feel the painful tissue. See if you can let it soften. If you are being treated, or are self-treating, and the tissue is softening, then you are doing exactly what you need to be doing. If the tissue is resisting, then you are putting too much pressure into the area. The body doesn't lie, so trust it.

When you feel pain or another sensation, try to acknowledge that sensation and then allow yourself to feel the tissue under it. Ask yourself some of the following questions. What does the tissue feel like? Is it hard or soft? Does it feel like a rock, a steel cable, a sponge, something else? Can I breathe into the area? Can I connect with that part of my body? Describe that area and picture it as clearly as you can. Then, give that area of your body permission to soften and see if you can feel the tissue changing.

See if you can notice even the smallest changes. If the tissue feels like a rock, try and imagine it slowly turning into clay or Jell-O. If you are being treated, see if you can picture and feel the therapist's hands sinking into your body. It may take some time to get this concept, especially if the area being treated has been painful and guarded for a long time. Don't be discouraged if initially you can't feel your body softening or changing. Just try some different visualizations every once in a while without overwhelming yourself. It may take several sessions before you become aware of any releases.

Being able to tune in and feel the release is an important part of the healing process. Feeling your body softening and releasing helps you know the body is doing what it needs to do to heal. The body will not release if it is being forced; it will not let itself be injured. This is an important concept to understand for self-treatment. When you feel your body softening—even a hair's width—then you know it's doing what it needs to do.

Try not to use pain as a guide during the release. We tend to think the pain should ease as a release occurs. This may be the case at times, but at other times the pain actually will get worse as the tissue releases. Why does this happen? The pain may intensify because as the outer layers release, you are now getting down to the key restrictions and these are sometimes the most painful areas.

When a spot being treated is uncomfortable, notice how you tense and mentally pull out of the area. Your breathing may become shallow at the same time. This is a natural response, so don't be hard on yourself when you feel the need to pull away from an uncomfortable sensation. Allow yourself to breathe fully into the area being treated and to feel every sensation as much as you can. You can use some of the preceding questions to help yourself bring more awareness into the area being treated.

As the layers are released, the pain can become intense, so you may feel yourself tensing. If you are having a hard time softening, ask your therapist for guidance. The therapist should be able to give you some tips that will help increase your awareness and release the tissue. After the therapist gives you some ideas, it will be up to you to quiet down and feel. Feeling is one of the key factors in allowing your body to heal.

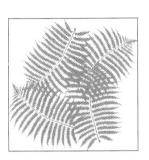

10

How do I bring in awareness and clear?

When you first hear your therapist suggest you "clear a space" or "let it go," you may not understand what she means. Doing an exercise that involves contracting and relaxing may help you understand these concepts. Try the following exercise and see if it helps.

Find a comfortable place to sit or lie down. Take a few breaths, let yourself become quiet, and feel your body soften. As you quiet down, let yourself become aware of an area in your body that feels tense or painful, or an area that is difficult to feel clearly.

Next, tighten that area and hold the tightness. Continue to increase the tightness in the area as much as you can without causing injury. As you hold this tension, feel the tightness fully and deeply. Also, feel the struggle in your body that results from your holding on to the tension when the body wants to let go. Then, take a deep breath and let go of the tension. Feel your body soften and let go of the tension in response. With each breath, let your body soften more and more.

This is what it's like to clear an area or allow the body to release. Most of the time, your body wants to soften, but the subconscious mind is telling it to stay tense. Your body may just need permission to let go, to stop guarding and protecting. Bringing awareness into a tight area is an important step in the healing process.

Often, feeling an area and breathing into it is all that is needed for that area to soften. Sometimes, some belief or fear is causing the tension or tightness. In these situations, you may feel emotions or have tissue memory come up. (See chapter 14, *Why are emotions coming up?*) Whatever the feeling is, allow yourself to feel it even more and give your body permission to do or feel whatever it needs to heal. Most of the time the body knows exactly what it needs to do; it just needs the mind to let go of control and allow the body heal.

Another approach that can help clear an area is breathing into the area that is tight or that is being treated. Try to breathe into the area the therapist's hands are touching. Sometimes it helps to visualize bringing a color or light into the area as the breath fills the area.

Just experiment and see what works for you. It may take some practice and you may need to try several different visualizations before you find one that works for you. Don't be hard on yourself! Remember most of us were taught not to feel, especially if the feeling involves pain or emotions. You may have difficulty at first with bringing awareness into your body. If you have been in pain for a long time it may be particularly difficult to allow yourself to feel uncomfortable sensations. Just be easy with yourself.

The more present and aware you are during the treatment, the better your results. When you find yourself struggling, remember letting go is no different than letting your breath out. It's a passive event. You just have to stop holding on and allow yourself to heal.

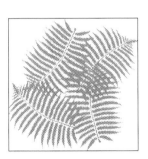

11

What do I do when I want to figure it out?

Sometimes we hinder our healing process because we think we need to know *why* we are feeling what we are feeling. Or, we think release would be more complete if what we are feeling "made sense." We can also hinder our healing process by trying to figure out what caused the pain, emotion, or restriction. When we are stuck in the mode of "figuring it out," we are actually limiting our ability to heal and let go. The truth is that if you really need to know the cause of what you're feeling, your body will let you know. Knowing why doesn't really need to be part of the healing process.

The following example illustrates how the healing process is often multi-faceted and overlapping. Let's say you fell and hit your head on a chair when you were 3; you crashed your bike at age 10; you had a car accident in your teens; you slipped on ice when you were in your

20s; and add in surgeries and other traumas that led you to the present moment. These traumas overlap each other and connect, like a three-dimensional spider web.

When one restriction is being released, it may trigger physical and emotional tissue memory from multiple traumas. You may feel fear from the car accident, pain from the bike wreck, anger from your surgeries, and so on. All of these feelings can mix together and won't make logical sense at all when they all come up at the same time. If you try to figure it out by trying to identify the *one thing* that is the source of all these feelings, you will limit yourself to healing only one of these traumas. If you can give up your need to know and instead just feel each sensation completely, you allow yourself to heal multiple traumas simultaneously.

There are times during a release when you will know the precise cause some of the sensations; at other times the sensations won't make any sense at all. Just allow yourself to feel whatever comes up. Let yourself be drawn down whatever path your body needs to take you. The body knows exactly what to do and how to take you where you need to go to heal.

I like to picture myself drifting down a river on a raft, just letting the river take me where it wants. Most of us have been trying to swim upstream because we thought we "knew" where we needed to go. Eventually, we get exhausted and we're forced to let the river take us where we need to go anyway. Why not just let yourself be guided from the beginning instead of waiting until you are broken down or exhausted?

The healing process does not need to be about struggling; it can be about learning to trust our inner guide and yielding instead of resisting. Let the healing process be as easy as possible. You have hurt, and tried to figure it out, long enough. If you could have figured it out, you would have done that by now. Let go, trust yourself, and allow yourself to heal.

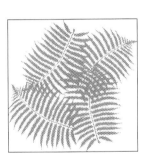

12

What if I was making progress but now I am having a flare up?

You are progressing along and then you have a flare up. The flare up could be a healing crisis—the process in which symptoms get worse before they get better. It can be very frustrating when this occurs, but it is often part of the healing process. This phase has to do with the mind/body connection or the mind/body communication. During this phase, the mind and the body are trying to learn how to communicate with each other again. Most of us have been taught we should ignore our insights, intuition, or inner guide. When we do start to reconnect by listening to our body or our inner wisdom, it's not always a smooth or easy transition. The following is an example of how the mind and then the body might interpret this "flare up."

Here's the mind's prospective:

"Here I am progressing along nicely with this myofascial release therapy. The body is finally starting to open up. I can feel the shifts; I am starting to feel good! The body is finally starting to let me do the things I want to do! Then, I do something I think is very insignificant, like walk 5 more minutes or do a few extra household chores, and—WHAM!—that crazy body has a full blown flare up. I even feel some symptoms that I haven't felt in months. What is up with that!?"

Now, let's look at this same situation from the body's perspective:

"Here I am finally starting to get some release from the restrictions that have been crushing me. Then, that crazy mind decided to push me more than normal and I got scared. Why? Because I am finally starting to make some progress and that darn mind is trying to force me to do something that feels bad again. I tried to be nice and just send the ache signal, but of course the mind just kept on pushing. Well, I have learned over time the only way to get the mind to stop is with a full blown sensory overload. In other words, I'm sending out the full alarm, the full pain signal. And since the mind didn't listen to the warning ache, I'm even going to send the alarm to some areas that haven't needed it for a while. I have to do this because I know the only way the mind will stop forcing me is if I really send out the pain signal. I am tired of being forced, I am ready to heal!"

Remember, over the years, most of us have learned to shut down the communication between mind and body. We are taught not to show emotions, to push through pain, to discount our intuition. In this state, pain is the only form of communication that can get our attention. And we've gotten so good at tuning out pain that it has to spread and become more intense to finally get our attention.

Through JFB-MFR treatments, we are starting to gain awareness and thereby learn to tune into the body. As this new communication begins, it can be a little fragile and sometimes pretty combustible. At times it might even seem like the mind and body are at war with each other. The mind feels the body let it down because the body can't do the things the mind wants to do. Sometimes we have lost almost all of our functional ability. The body feels the mind has let it down because the mind keeps forcing the body to do things that hurt.

It's going to take time before these two systems trust each other again. In the process, there may be battles for control, with each side returning to what is familiar. For the mind, reverting to the familiar will be forcing through the pain. For the body, it will be sending out the full alarm to get the mind to stop. Mind and body will each tend to revert to those things which helped enable survival in the past. Emotions may also surface—feelings of anger, betrayal, guilt, etc. The only way the body will start trusting the mind to take care of it again will be by the actions we take. When the body starts sending out the subtle signals, do we listen to them or ignore them? Do we take time to self-treat and really give our full attention to the body?

As this communication improves, trust is established and the body won't need to send the full alarms. The body will start sending more subtle messages—like pressure or tightness—and the mind will now be open enough to feel these sensations and use them for guidance. Again, the key is feeling—specifically, feeling without judgment, feeling the sensations fully and letting them guide us where to go next. This may mean doing self-treatment, journaling, or feeling an emotion that has been ignored. In turn, we will be able to increase functional activities and do so with less pain and more ease. We will start to return to a fun and fulfilling life style!

Embrace the struggles and remember to feel the sensations. Both sides in the battle—mind and body—feel they have been wronged and both need some love, forgiveness, and healing. The end result definitely will be worth it.

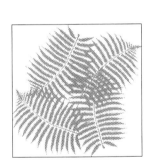

13

What if I have leveled out?

As you have probably heard or experienced for yourself, progression is not linear with JFB-MFR. As described in chapter 7 on symptoms changing and in chapter 12 on flare ups and symptoms increasing, sometimes it can seem like you take two steps forward and then one step back. You may even reach a plateau where your progress seems to stop, to level out, for a while. This might happen for a variety of reasons. The following suggestions might help you progress to the next level of healing.

1. **Treat places in your body you do not normally treat**. Sometimes we get into a routine of treating where we *think* we should treat. As we progress in JFB-MFR, the body will shift and change. This means places that used to have the most significant restrictions have released, and now other places

in the body need treatment. Take out all your self-treatment exercises and treat your entire body. Do some self-unwinding and let your body tell you where you need to be treated.

2. **Whenever you are aware of the fact that you have leveled out or are "stuck," let yourself feel whatever comes up.** You may need to feel and release emotions to progress to the next level in your healing process. Let yourself feel any anger, frustration, sadness, etc. that may come up while you aware of leveling out; see where feeling and releasing such emotions leads you.

3. **Write in your journal.** Writing in your journal can be a very effective method for tapping into your subconscious mind and leading you to your next level of healing. Following are some topics you could address in your journal.

   • Remember another time in your life when you have felt this way.

   • Start a sentence with "Right now I feel…" and just see where this takes you.

   • Consider what you are gaining from holding onto this pain or sensation. (Sometimes we become so used to having a pain or a sensation that it can actually be frightening to let it go; holding onto it may be painful but it is familiar.

Be open as you consider this topic and do not judge whatever answer comes up. Considering this topic is just another way to increase your awareness and to clear another level for further healing.)

4. **Get treatment from another therapist.** At the treatment centers, we treat as a team of therapists. Every therapist brings a unique style to treatment and you may need a variety of styles during the treatment process. Getting treatment by a variety of therapists is a very good way to receive all the aspects of treatment you need. You might even find you develop a sense for when treatment from a particular therapist would benefit you the most.

5. **Increase the amount of treatment you are receiving.** When you reach a restriction that has been in place for a long time, you may need to increase the amount of treatment you receive in order to get to the core of that restriction. Once you get to the core layer of a restriction, it will release completely; until then, the restriction often tightens back down between sessions. This is why the intensive program at one of the MFR centers is so powerful and effective: your body doesn't have time to tighten back down between sessions and you are likely to be able to get to some of your core restrictions.

6. **Reread John's book and watch his videos.** John's book *Healing Ancient Wounds: The Renegade's Wisdom,* and his *Fireside Chat* and MFR series videos, each have deep insights that can help you along your healing journey. The book you are reading now just touches on the basics; John's book and videos are invaluable during your treatment process. Reading and rereading his book, and viewing and reviewing the video, are priceless.

7. **Read other books on the healing process.** I have written another book called *Feeling Your Way Through.* It is more comprehensive than this one and will be helpful as you progress along your healing journey. You may also be drawn to other books to help you along the way. Peter Levine's *Waking the Tiger* and Colin Tipin's *Radical Forgiveness* are books that can be very helpful in the healing process. Authors of other books that may help are: Wayne Dyer, Caroline Myss, Don Miguel Ruiz, and Lee Coit, to name just a few. There is a wealth of information out there. Go with the books that feel right to you.

8. **Take a break from getting treatment.** Sometimes you just need to sit with what you feel and see where that takes you. This often prompts you to feel some sensations you may have been trying to avoid.

These are suggestions to help you along. The truth is that each person's healing process is unique. The key is tuning into your own guide and picking the path that feels right for you.

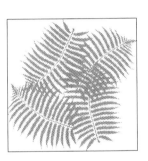

14

Why are emotions coming up?

During a treatment, all kinds of sensations and feelings can be released. This includes shaking, tremors, pain, and emotions. Why does this happen? This can occur when tissue memory is triggered during a release.

Tissue memory is a natural and normal occurrence. Consider this example. Remember a time when you had the flu or were very sick. What happened the next time you smelled or tasted the kind food you ate just before you got sick? Typically, you had some sort of physical response to that smell or taste. Your stomach may have gotten queasy, you may have started to sweat, and you may have even come close to throwing up.

Your body was having a physical response to a memory. Your body associates the smell or taste of that food with becoming sick and it doesn't want to be sick like that again. To try to prevent you from getting sick again, the next time you smelled or tasted that food, your body reminded you of how sick you had been the last time you smelled or tasted that food.

When this happens, the body is having a response to a proprioceptive trigger. Proprioception involves the five senses: sight, smell, taste, sound, and touch. When any of these receptors is triggered, tissue memory can occur too, as in the preceding example.

Another reaction most people can relate to is having a memory associated with a song (i.e., reacting to the sound proprioceptor). You hear a certain song and you are "taken back" to a particular time in your life. Maybe it's a song you heard at a wedding, a funeral, or prom. As you remember the event, you may also feel emotions associated with that event.

When the fascia is released through touch (which is one of the proprioceptors), tissue memory may be triggered in the process. If an area being released was injured during a scary event—car accident, abuse, etc.—sensations that occurred during that event might also be released. You might feel fear; your body might shake; you might feel the pain just as intensely as when the trauma originally occurred. You might feel any and all of the sensations that were caused during the trauma and that have been trapped in the fascia, and in your body. You are actually becoming aware of what your body is feeling all the time on the subconscious level. When this happens, what you need to do is feel *fully* the sensations that occurred during the trauma so they can be released from your body.

Feeling these sensations *fully* is easy to say, but not necessarily easy to do. Remember the sensations can feel as intense as they did during the initial trauma itself. Many times the sensations that occurred were overwhelming, which is why we weren't able to release them in the first place. When we are overwhelmed with pain, fear, etc., one of our automatic self-defense mechanisms is to leave our body. To "leave the body" is to become completely numb, pushing the pain and emotions below the conscious level.

When the tissue memory is triggered, the sensations that arise can be just as overwhelming as they were in the original trauma. Remember you don't have to feel it all at once. Just allow yourself to feel as much you can and then pull out of the feeling if it begins to be overwhelming. It's okay to chip away at it bit by bit. You always have the control over how much you feel. Also, remember to tell yourself the traumatic event is over and you survived it. Tell yourself it is okay to feel and release now so you can live fully in the present. It's time to let yourself heal.

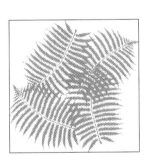

15

Why would I want to feel the emotions that come up?

Emotions often surface during the treatment process. In fact, feeling the emotions can be a very big catalyst in the healing process. Why is it important to tap into and feel any emotions associated with our pain or injury? As we all know, stress and emotions can cause physical tightness and pain. Don't confuse this phenomenon with the notion that your pain is "just in your head" and discounting it as such. The physical restrictions caused by physical *and emotional* traumas and stresses are real. They can be seen and felt, and they can cause crushing pain.

Almost every kind of chronic and acute pain has an emotional component. The emotional component might be fear or anger that occurred at the time of injury, or frustration and sense of loss of control that often accompanies chronic pain. If the emotional component isn't addressed, then the physical restriction will not release fully, causing continued pain.

As emotional pain comes to the surface, we may wonder why we would want to feel those awful feelings. Why not just stuff them down? Beside the fact that you will not be pain-free if you hold on to the emotions, you will not truly live until the emotions are cleared. These stored emotions are the cause our strong reactions to certain triggers. A reaction is just what it says: a re-action. When you fly off the handle, or start crying for no apparent reason, you are reacting to emotions that are stuffed inside. You are trapped in the past, unable to truly live in the moment.

All of this became clear and real to me after I finally cleared the pain surrounding my dad's death. Before I did this, whenever I would think of my dad, all I could feel and remember was the pain and grief surrounding his loss. I didn't want to think or talk about my dad because I would feel those feelings of sadness and grief. Now that I've cleared these pains, I can tap into and feel all the love and good times we shared.

When I cleared the pain and sorrow I was holding onto from the death of my dad, I was able to reconnect with the love I shared with him. By clearing our restrictions and letting go of the pain of the past, we can embrace fully the love and beauty of the present. The process may not always be easy, but it is always worth it.

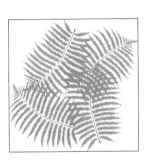

16

What if I don't want to feel or remember that again?

Most of us say we don't want to feel the pain "again," or we have already "dealt with that" and don't want to remember it again. If you have truly "dealt with" an issue, truly healed, then it will no longer cause a reaction in your body when you talk or think about it. When you start to talk or think about an event, if your body starts to tighten or if tears come up, then more healing needs to occur.

Most of us have been taught you process past pain and trauma by talking about them. This only deals with *part* of the healing process; it's why people can go to talk therapy for years and still not "resolve" their issues. You will heal truly only when you connect fully to your mind and body, allowing yourself to feel the pain and the other sensations associated with the trauma and then letting go of all those sensations.

The fact is, on the subconscious level, you experience unresolved trauma all day and all night long, like a broken record. To your subconscious mind, the trauma is happening continuously. You feel the truck is about to hit you; the surgical knife is cutting you; the abuse is still going on.

In the safety of the therapeutic environment, it is better to feel intense therapeutic pain, sadness, anger, or other sensations and emotions for a short time, then to spend the rest of your life "coping" with any of these. "Coping" is a losing battle; it is simply your subconscious mind controlling you by bracing constantly against the unresolved trauma. This constant bracing causes the ground substance of the fascia to solidify, which in turn forms restrictions. The constant subconscious bracing worsens, spreading the restrictions, and therefore the symptoms, throughout your body over time. The end result is you feel like you are wearing a straitjacket or are totally numb inside and out.

JFB-MFR never injures or re-traumatizes. JFB-MFR allows for the discovery of unresolved physical/emotional trauma. The mind/body is then able to process this information through the conscious mind and complete the process known as release. JFB-MFR allows for healing on the deepest level.

Remember, you don't have to feel it all at once. Each time you allow yourself to feel the pain/trauma deeply and then clear (release) it, you come closer to healing fully. Each time you do this, you will become lighter and become more yourself again. You are always in control and can choose to feel as much or as little as you are ready to do at the time. As you chip away a little at a time, you will begin to feel the changes as they occur. This will then help you trust both your body and the healing process and you will be able to feel more and more deeply. The more you allow yourself to feel, the more quickly you will be able to heal.

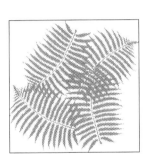

17

Why is my body moving?

Remember your body is like a three-dimensional web of connected tissue. Fascia is not linear and neither are releases. As the restrictions begin to release, movement might start to occur; this is called unwinding. Sometimes unwinding occurs in small, subtle motions and movements, and at other times, the unwinding can involve the entire body. Whether the movement is small or large, you might have powerful tissue memory and emotions come up. During any session, you might shift back and forth between being still and having very energized unwindings.

Unwinding is your body's way of putting a part (shoulder, leg, head, etc.), or all, of the body in the position in which the injury occurred. Moving into such a position helps your body to achieve a complete release. For example, if you hurt your arm while throwing a ball, your arm might move itself over your head in an unwinding until it reaches the position it was in when it was injured during the throw. Or, you might have been thrown from a horse and landed upside down. In that case, your body may actually need to reproduce the motion of the fall to release that trauma.

During an unwinding, your body will move until it gets back into the position of injury; that position is called a "still point." Your body will wait in this position, processing in whatever manner it needs to do. This might be through letting out emotions, through a physical response like shaking or sweating, or even through a feeling of calm. Once this still point is resolved, you will move on to the next layer or position. Strong tissue memory often comes up during unwinding. You might have sensations come up that occurred during the trauma, as I explained in the chapter on tissue memory (see chapter 14, *Why are emotions coming up?*).

After that restriction is resolved, your body will move on to the next still point. This next still point may be completely different from the previous one; however, the body might return to the exact same position it was just in while you release at a deeper level. If the restriction was due to a very traumatic event, you might need to unwind several times to allow for a full release. It might be too painful or scary to feel all the sensations associated with the trauma at once.

Every night while we sleep, the body naturally releases some of the traumas through dreaming and movement. The only problem is that the bed gets in the way! This is why you need the assistance of a skilled therapist to help you with the process. The therapist's job is to help take gravity out of the system and provide a safe environment for you to release. The therapist does not lift or move you; he just follows wherever the body leads and helps you stay in still points until they fully release.

As with any part of the JFB-MFR treatment, the best advice is to "let go of the outcome." Let each unwinding be whatever it needs to be, whether it manifests as subtle (small) movements or as more energetic (full body) movements. Remember both subtle and energetic movements are perfect; one is not better than the other. Sometimes we think we need to have big motion and a lot of noise to have a powerful unwinding. That is simply not true. Sometimes, while the body stays completely still, a very powerful unwinding occurs internally. Unwinding is more about letting go than about "getting there."

Always let go of any expectations before your treatment. Give yourself permission to do and feel whatever you need to do to reach your next level of healing. At the time of treatment, your body might need unwinding with an emotional release, or structural work, or any number of other things. Trust that your body knows what it needs and take all the pressure off yourself. If you let go in this way, you will end up getting exactly the treatment you need.

18
Can I treat myself?

One of the best things about JFB-MFR is that you can treat yourself. You actually can have a major impact on your own recovery. In fact, your therapist can only take them so far, and then it's up to you. JFB-MFR is an interactive treatment. You need to be aware and present during treatments—as discussed in preceding chapters—and the more you self-treat, the more quickly you can progress.

- *How do you know where to treat?*

    You can treat places where you feel symptoms and also places your therapist suggests you treat. Remember that where you feel the symptoms may be different from where the cause of the problem is located. Ask your therapist the location of some of your key areas to treat and ask how to treat those areas. I always tell my patients that if they don't know where to treat, they should just ask the body. Just reach over your head and start moving and stretching like you do when you wake up in the morning. Move your body and see how it feels. You will be able to feel where you are tight or where you have pain and that is your body's way of telling you where to treat. Start becoming aware of how your body feels throughout the day. This will guide you to areas that need to be treated.

- *How do I treat myself?*

Your therapist should be able to direct you in stretches and in the use of tools for self-treatment. We usually have patients use the following tools: small ball, foam roll, Nola Rola, Theracane, and Occipivot. With these tools, you can pretty much treat your entire body. The tools are a great investment and will more than pay for themselves with the relief they provide. You can purchase all of these tools directly from the manufacturer or you can order them from the Myofascial Release Treatment Center (1-800-327-2425). You can also order John's DVD *Myofascial Freedom* from either of his Malvern clinic or his Sedona clinic. This video goes over self-treatment techniques.

The book *Myofascial Stretching: A Guide to Self-treatment*, by Brenda Pardy, OTR and Jill Morton, MS, OTR, is a very good resource for self-treatment. This book has detailed pictures of stretches and the use of the small ball for self-treatment; it also has some very good general information on self-treatment. You can order it by going to www.DenverMyofascialRelease.com or calling 1-303-649-9007. *Comprehensive Myofascial Self Treatment,* by Joyce Karnis Patterson, PT, is another good resource for self-treatment. To order this book, visit www.mfrselftreat.com

• *How do I know if I'm doing it right?*

This calls for awareness on your part. Just like during a treatment, when you are self-treating, you need to feel the area you are treating and feel the releases when they happen. As you know, sometimes it can be painful when a restriction is being treated. Whenever you are treating a restriction, breathe into the area and feel what the tissue is doing (see chapter 9, *What does my therapist mean by "feel under the pain"?*). As long as the tissue is softening and giving—no matter how small the change—you are doing what your body needs. If your body is resisting, you are putting too much pressure into the area. Forcing the system will only cause more tightness to occur.

- *How long do I treat myself?*

  Remember it takes a minimum of 120 seconds for a release to *start* happening. You should hold the release for at least 3–5 minutes. Anything less will be a waste of time. While self-treating, don't look at the clock continuously, as doing so will distract you from really feeling any release that occurs. Put on some calming music and hold a release for at least one composition. That way you know you are holding the release long enough.

- *How often should I treat?*

  Self-treatment should become part of your daily routine. You don't need to treat every area every day. As you become aware of the significant areas, you will realize where you need to focus your attention. Consider your predominant posture during a typical day; this will point you to where you need to focus some treatment. Most people need to open up their chest and their hip flexors because they spend a lot of time sitting, driving, typing, etc. and these activities keep them in a flexed position.

- *What if I am sore after I treat myself?*

  As long as you were treating yourself with awareness and not forcing the system, you did exactly what the body needed. As with treatment from your therapist, you may have soreness or even experience a healing crisis after a self-treatment session. If you did force the system, then you gave yourself a traditional treatment and you will have only temporary results.

The more you put into your self-treatment program, the more you will get out of it and better you will feel. JFB-MFR teaches you how to take care of yourself for the rest of your life. It helps you maintain a functional and pain free lifestyle; self-treatment is a critical part of this maintenance.

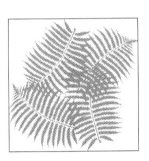

19

What about diet and supplements and JFB-MFR?

The following questions come up frequently. What diet will help the JFB-MFR process? Would a vegetarian diet be beneficial? Should I avoid carbohydrates? What supplements should I take?

When these questions are asked in seminars, John makes this point: it is more important to establish a system that can actually absorb nutrients than it is to put nutrients into a system that is full of restrictions. Spending money on the best supplement—or following the most recent anti-aging/cleansing diet—will not do any good if your system is too restricted to process these nutrients.

Fascia goes all the way down to the cellular level; it is what gives the cell its shape. Actually, the restrictions can be preventing the nutrients from getting into the cells. The nutrients are already in the body, but the cells are clamped down and unable to process them.

When considering diet and supplements, be aware of the terms "organic," "natural," and "homeopathic." Sometimes people feel using "natural" supplements means there can be no harmful side effects. Or, they believe anything "organic," "natural," or "homeopathic" is intrinsically good for them. Anything used to mask symptoms, instead of helping the body correct itself, is simply something used to treat the symptoms; it doesn't matter if it's natural or synthetic. The purity of a supplement is irrelevant when the body is unable to process the supplement due to restrictions.

If you are considering taking a supplement or medicine, do your research first. Natural and organic products have just as much potential to cause side effects as do synthetic and conventional products. It's best to know about those things *before* you start using a product. When someone advises you use a product, consider the person's training, education, experience, and expertise. Remember, it is okay to ask questions and to think for yourself.

The biggest factor in establishing and maintaining health is opening up the system. When the body is free of restrictions, it can heal itself. Until then, no matter what you put in your body, it's like pouring water on a rock; nothing will be absorbed into the system.

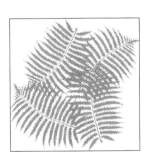

20

What about exercising?

During the treatment process, questions frequently come up about when to start exercising and what exercises to do. What I'm going to provide here are the basic guidelines that will coincide with your progression during JFB-MFR treatments.

I tell my patients to hold off on any strengthening or stabilization exercises during the beginning phases of JFB-MFR. Why? Because strengthening and stabilization exercises you do before your body is balanced will only further your problem. In other words, you are strengthening in a position of dysfunction.

It is very important to hold off on any trunk stabilization exercises until the pelvis is balanced and stays that way. This includes all Pilates, crunches, sit ups, etc. If you are really into fitness, you may have a hard time with this idea at first. However, once you have felt an intense psoas release, you probably won't want to have the psoas released again—that will likely lead you to be more willing to stick to this guideline!

As you become more aware of the restricted places in your body, you can start exercising *with awareness.* This means if you are exercising an area with significant restrictions, you maintain the awareness needed to notice if you are strengthening or straining the restricted area. If you are straining the area, you should either stop doing that particular exercise or perform self-treatment to that area once you are done with the exercise. This will help prevent the area from becoming more restricted.

Awareness is the key. It's all about developing communication between the mind and the body. You may be one of the many people who have learned to tune out or push through pain or discomfort. Now, you are being asked to notice pain and discomfort and to be willing to stop doing an activity when you feel either one. Doing this can be a very difficult at first, so ask your therapist to help with this concept (See chapter 9, *What does my therapist mean by "feel under the pain"?*).

Another aspect to consider is the reason behind your need to exercise. Many people use exercise as a way to "burn off the stress." Many people have flat out said they couldn't stop running, biking, etc. or they would "go crazy." They admit exercise is their way to deal with the stress in their lives. If they stopped exercising, then they would have to feel. Guess what, that is exactly what you need to do—you need to feel! Let yourself feel whatever it is you are trying to avoid. Then, release the feelings instead of stuffing them down or burning them off with exercise.

There is a difference between exercising to feel better and exercising to control feelings and emotions. Changing or limiting your exercise routine can cause some chaos. If this happens, it is very important to let yourself feel whatever comes up so you can release it. (See chapters 14 and 15, *Why are emotions coming up?* and *Why would I want to feel the emotions that come up?*)

You should know you will be able to return to your normal exercise program again. This break in your exercise program is necessary to give your body time to open up and balance out. The goal is for you to return to the same or an even higher level of activity with less discomfort and with more ease.

Ask your therapist to show you self-treatment exercises that specifically help release the tight areas that either prevent you from exercising or cause you to tighten down even further. This way you will take an active role in your recovery process and in your return to exercising. The more proactive you become in your healing process, the more quickly you will progress.

21

Can JFB-MFR help prevent surgery?

Some people arrive at our treatment center having been told surgery is the only way to improve their condition. Many of these same people have already had multiple, unsuccessful surgeries and want to avoid repeating that experience. People also call to ask if JFB-MFR can prevent the need for surgery. The answer is the same to everyone: If the situation is an emergency, get the surgery! If it's not an emergency, try JFB-MFR first. What have you got to lose?

No one can know before treatment whether JFB-MFR will prevent the need for non-emergency surgery. However, during or after treatment, it is not unusual to find the pain, restricted motion, or other symptoms have subsided or disappeared completely and such surgery is no longer needed. This scenario is most frequent with conditions in which doctors are unable to determine the source of the pain or other symptoms, but they "think surgery should help."

Having JFB-MFR treatment before non-emergency surgery can help in a couple of ways. First, treatment may help decrease the pain. Pain often occurs because the body is being compressed. Remember, a fascial restriction can have the tensile strength of up to 2000 pounds of per square inch. A force of this strength can literally crush structures in the body, producing almost every symptom in the body, including nerve and joint pain.

Second, having treatment will help open up your body, and the more open your body is before surgery, the faster your recovery. Most people have tightness and restrictions *prior* to surgery. With the effects of new scar tissue formed *after* surgery, the body becomes even tighter, and this can make recovery from surgery even more painful and difficult. Eliminating tightness and restrictions before surgery can help tissue heal much more quickly.

Joint replacement is a prime example of the kind of non-emergency surgery I've just described. Think of this situation in terms of your car needing a front-end alignment. If your car's tires are wearing unevenly, you know the alignment is off. If you just replace the tires without fixing the alignment, the new tires will just wear unevenly again. So, it makes sense to bring the car into alignment before installing new tires. Actually, having JFB-MFR prior to a joint replacement may eliminate the need for the joint replacement. After treatment, if you still need the replacement, your body will be in alignment. This will help the new joint last longer and help you heal with fewer problems. (As an example of how much force restrictions can cause, imagine the pressure—and the misalignment it causes—that wears out the metal components comprised by an artificial joint!)

Why not try JFB-MFR first? It can't hurt and you have only some restrictions to lose!

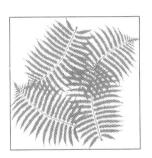

22

Why doesn't my therapist want family members or friends in the treatment room?

To enable you to benefit fully from the treatment process, your therapist generally discourages having family members or friends in the treatment room with you. It can be very hard to let go completely when a family member or friend is in the room. Belief systems might be limiting your healing and sometimes such belief systems were created by your family dynamics. Having a family member or friend in the room can prevent you from feeling and expressing your pain or emotions fully.

Under some circumstances, the therapist allows a family member to observe treatment to see what is involved in the process. This is generally only when a minor is being treated. In such cases, the therapist works to establish treatment as soon as possible without the family member present.

We want each person to have the treatment held as sacred space, without any fear of judgment. Some aspect of your signs and symptoms might be tied into something involving your family or friends, or into an area of your life which you do not feel comfortable sharing with your family or friends. In such cases, you might feel very uneasy letting go while others are in the room. You might not even be aware you are holding back until you have the chance to be alone.

If family or friends want to be in the room, but you feel you would benefit more by having the treatment alone, you can have your therapist talk with them. The more they are educated in the JFB-MFR process, the more supportive they can be of your growth. To help them better understand JFB-MFR, you could suggest they watch John's video *The Fireside Chat* or read his book *Healing Ancient Wounds: The Renegade's Wisdom*.

Creating a healing environment for you is essential to your treatment. This is your healing process, so give yourself the chance to benefit as much as possible.

23

JFB-MFR:
Motion for Life!

As you progress through treatment, you may find yourself asking your therapist questions like the following. "When will I be free of all restrictions?" "How long do I need to do the self-treatment?" "When am I done?" "Do I have to do this forever?" Think of it this way: do you only brush your teeth two or three times a week for two months and expect your teeth to stay healthy for the rest of your life?

Most of us have come to understand we need to brush and floss our teeth at least twice a day to promote healthy teeth and gums. This has become a habit, so it doesn't seem like anything out of the ordinary. But when a therapist suggests doing something every day to promote a healthy body, many people get upset.

A daily regimen of oral self-treatment—brushing and flossing your teeth—tends to keep teeth and gums healthy and pain-free. Similarly, a daily regimen of bodily self-treatment—including JFB-MFR techniques—tends to keep the body healthy and pain-free. As you get into a pattern of treating yourself, self-treatment will become just as much of a habit as brushing and flossing your teeth. If you are in pain, you'll develop the habit of grabbing the small ball, foam roll, or Theracane instead of the Advil. This is what your therapist means by "tapping into your inner power and taking care of yourself." As you get into the habit of treating your body, you will begin to understand where to treat to help keep yourself feeling good.

When you get into the habit of treating yourself, you will actually feel out of sorts when you don't treat yourself daily. It will be like going a few days without brushing your teeth. Your body and mind begin to crave the treatment because it just feels right. It feels so good to release the restrictions that develop over the course of a day.

Your body undergoes a lot of stress and strain every day just doing normal activities such as sitting, driving, using the computer, and lifting. Treating every day helps deter minor aches and pains from developing into major ones. Daily self-treatment also gives you time to process whatever mental stress may have occurred during the day. It becomes a time to just "chill out" and do something good for yourself.

JFB-MFR gives you the tools you need not only to restore your function, but also to live an overall more fulfilling life—the tools for Motion for Life!!

Afterword

At his seminars, John likes to say "Life is motion" and JFB-MFR can help you regain and maintain a healthy and pain-free lifestyle. I couldn't agree more, especially since it was JFB-MFR that helped give me my life back. This is why my treatment center is called Motion for Life. My hope is this book will help other people become more aware of JFB-MFR so each can get his or her life back too.

I hope this book will help you along your journey to a healthy and happy life. As more questions come up, remember you can ask them on John's chat line at: www.myofascialrelease.com. The chat line is a great resource for support and a way to connect with therapists or patients in your area.

If you have any questions, feel free to contact me through my website at www.motionforlife.net. Here's to living an active and adventurous life!